Also by Patricia Betty

Aromatherapy: A Scented Journey by Patricia Betty and Nancy Schenck

Aromatherapy: A Personal Journey Through Your Senses (audiotape)

5/94

Linda, It's a great pleasure
to see you again!
Hope all your journeys
are scented & pleasant!
Pat Betty

Aromatherapy

a personal journey through your senses

A Workbook

by Patricia Betty

Published in the United States by Pebble Publications
c/o E-Scentially Yours, Ltd.

ISBN 0-9641205-4-2

Cover art and original illustrations by Carol Goebel.
Cover and book design by Zí Design.

This book is dedicated to the return journey home.

acknowledgments

To my clients and students, my editor Amelia Sheldon, the Tawfiks, Hattie Wiener, Marie Zazzi and Superfoot, Sally, Susan and Calvin. To my helpful and willing reader, Laura Pavan. To the wonderful people who helped with creative and timely production, Adrian Westney, Jr. (Audio); Roger Smith, Jr., Diane Baier and Bill G. Neely of Zí Design (Graphics); and Carol Goebel (Original Artwork). Thanks for the encouraging words and support.

Aromatherapy

A Personal Journey Through Your Senses

A Workbook

introduction

My goal in writing this book is to introduce you to the process of viewing the plants and the essential oils that are used in aromatherapy in a deep and personal way. I call this process interactive viewing. Through it you examine elements of each plant and oil while keeping your own personal reaction to their effects upon all of your senses in mind. Throughout the workbook I will offer suggestions and gently guide you through a selection of plants from the aromatherapist's garden, asking you to imagine the appearance, feel and smell of each plant as it appears in nature. There is a drawing of each plant and a sample of the essential oil extracted from it to make your experience of each plant more tangible.

I hope the exercises here will not only allow you to enjoy each plant and oil a little more fully, but will also leave an imprint of each of them upon all of your senses. Hopefully, these imprints will deepen your understanding of each plant and help you to apply and combine the oils for the most effective remedies possible.

This workbook can be used as an extension of my seminars and workshops, as an accompaniment to my first book AROMATHERAPY: A SCENTED JOURNEY, or as a unique experience in and of itself.

What if you slept?

And what if, in your sleep, you dreamed?

And what if, in your dream, you went to heaven and there plucked
a beautiful flower?

And what if, when you awoke, you had the flower in your hand?

Ah, what then?

— Samuel Taylor Coleridge

Aromatherapy

a personal journey through your senses

In order to fully know the plants that provide essential oils, we must first become aware of the many ways that we have of experiencing them. This first exercise will help to reacquaint you with your own senses. Treat it as a guided meditation. You may want to read it over once and then break it into sections, completing each sense exploration before moving on to the next one.

* * * *

Close your eyes. Sit back comfortably. Relax. Breathe deeply and slowly and let us begin our journey.

Focus on the sensations you feel. What sense kicks in most, it is our ***hearing***. You might begin to hear your own or another person's breathing, other noises in the room, or even the wriggling of your body.

Keep your eyes closed and try to consciously awaken your other senses. Hard isn't it? Don't be discouraged. We rely primarily on our eyesight to give us cues in our world. With eyes closed, you probably are very aware that your sense of ***hearing*** is a close second to that of *sight.*

After exploring these two senses, you may be at a loss when trying to identify the next strongest sense you feel. Let me guide you a bit. Reach up and touch your hair, then touch the back of your neck, your face, your

clothes, and your arms. By doing this, you are unlocking your ***sense of touch*** (or tactile sense). What do these areas feel like? Go back (eyes still closed) and repeat this touching exercise. Note the various textures of your own skin and hair. Could you describe what you feel? Think about the words you would use to describe each new section of your body as you run your hands slowly over it. Commit these sensations to memory.

Now reach for a piece of candy or fruit. Sniff it carefully, then put it into your mouth. Roll it around your tongue, savor it, then chew it slowly and carefully — enjoying its taste, then swallow. The actual taste, or the memory of luscious-tasting food or drink, can almost instantly trigger our salivary glands to respond. The memory of taste can also set off another vital sense very closely linked to taste — ***the sense of smell.***

Open your eyes.

As part of this exercise, I would like you to explore a few very distinct scents including vinegar, honey, peanut butter, a lemon, ordinary aspirin, cloves, nutmeg, alcohol, and perfume. You can do this exercise at home with any variety of ordinary household items. Inhale the aroma of each item carefully, as if you were smelling it for the first time. Commit the nuances of each object's scent to memory. Breathe deeply in between each substance you smell. How do the scents compare to each other? Take your time. Make this a slow, languorous experience. Try putting one of the substances on your skin and experiencing the effect of it there while inhaling the blended scent of it with that of your skin. This is a helpful exercise to return to time and again.

Now, get up and stretch for a bit. Shake your body out; loosen your shoulder and neck joints, wiggle your arms, legs, and hips. Bend from the waist and let your torso and arms hang loosely over your feet. This will help you to relax your spine.

We will now delve into two other senses that contribute to a more subtle awareness of your surroundings than any of your other senses.

Sit down and close your eyes again.

I would like to make you more aware of your sense of ***proprioception.*** Proprioception is the awareness of mass in relation to space. All of our cells and systems have this awareness of how they relate to their neighbors.

To get in touch with your proprioception, tune your attention inward, onto your body. Relax and try to feel how your muscles hang from and are connected to your bones. Become aware of how your posture affects your muscles — slump and straighten.

Turn your head, touch your ear down to your shoulder, notice how your sense of balance changes. Close your eyes and bring your arm straight up in front of your body. Follow the movement of your arm with your proprioceptive sense — feel the relationship of your hand and arm to the rest of your body and to space in general.

Gently move your arms and then your entire body — imagine you are a harem dancer, undulate that arm and follow the movements with your feeling sense. Have fun with this new awareness! This sense is a close kin to your intuitive sense.

Now, sit completely motionless. I want you to become aware of the charge that your body emits even when you are still. Hold the flat of your palm about 2 inches above your forearm. Increase the space between your palm and arm by raising the palm about another 2 inches. Feel the tingling warmth of your electrical aura — the vibrational current that you give off. Trace this warmth up and down your whole arm. Try it over your heart, the other arm, your face, legs, etc. Pay close attention, the warmth will be greater in some areas than it is in others. All things have this vibrational current caused by atomic movement. Try to tune into this invisible field and recognize it in all living things around you.

Now that you have a keen awareness of all your senses, open your eyes. Really look around at all that surrounds you — the familiar and the unfamiliar. Notice the appeal of various objects. Try to see beauty in that which you hadn't before —maybe in the perfection of a lemon's shape, the caramel color of honey, or the contour of a bottle. Try to retain this openness to beauty in all of its forms as you go through your life. It will provide you with many unexpected treasures.

Breathe deeply and embrace your heightened sense of awareness as you begin your journey into the scented land — the world of aromatherapy.

preface

Since my introduction to the organized world of aromatherapy 17 years ago, I have tried to notice the interrelationships among all living things and to bring this new awareness to my aromatherapy practice. I have never lost that certain awe and respect that I had upon the discovery of the complexities of the atomic structure and the undefinable, invisible "force" that propels what we call life in plants and animals.

Ponder for a minute, if you will, the ceaseless movement of the atoms that come together to form our bodies. Similar atoms also move in the plants that nourish us, give us oxygen, and provide a feast of beauty for our eyes. Elements of these plants supply products that house us, make the paper we are holding, provide our medicines, and a host of other things we daily take for granted. They provide the beautiful aromatic scents that can so uplift us and enhance the quality of our lives! I call this ceaseless movement of atoms the "dance of life".

Scented molecules escape from plants by doing a dance of their own. The atomic molecules of the particular scent break off the plant and go back out into the air, or "evaporate". This evaporation, which is what has happened when we actually perceive the scent, can sometimes approach us in wave-like rhythms.

* * * *

This is an aromatherapy journey, and therefore we will focus our attention mainly on the scented essential oil molecules and the host plants that create them. However, your understanding will be that much deeper if you

approach this subject with the *heightened* awareness that comes from the use of all of your senses and a knowledge and respect of the interconnectedness of all life.

The predominant green color of our earth is produced, as we know, by the ingredient chlorophyll that is made by plants. Chlorophyll (very similar in makeup to our own blood) is the ingredient that plants use to trap sunlight. The plants use that stored light energy to make food and other organic compounds.

Since we cannot directly eat sunlight or directly convert sunlight into food for our bodies, we humans and other animals depend on the sunlight that plants have trapped and stored in various edible forms such as starch, fruit, seeds, nuts, and leaves.

We humans have named the production of chlorophyll and oxygen by plants their "primary system". A "secondary system" also operates concurrently in plants. This "secondary system" makes complex storage items that we consider medicinal compounds and includes essential oils and other extracts. Some of these medicinal compounds which can be found in essential oils are: medicinal alcoholic terpene; intoxicating alcohols, such as ethyl alcohol (which helps explain the uplifting, euphoric feeling after an aromatherapy treatment or upon constant inhalation of the oils); citric acids; analgesics; salicylic acid (the basis of aspirin); and many others too numerous to mention here.

These essential oils can play a dramatic role in how we feel, physically and psychologically. They can be applied to the skin directly or introduced to

our hormone glands through inhalation or topical application (like bathing or massage). Tactile application of oils makes the skin silky, more lubricated, visibly cleaner and increases the receptivity of the nerve endings there. Deep inhalation or prolonged application of oils can change our moods and increase the production of certain hormones. For example, some oils induce the body to release endorphins that relax the brain, others cause cortisone to be emitted to help decrease inflammation.

In our book AROMATHERAPY: A SCENTED JOURNEY, Nancy Schenck and I discuss the role aromatherapy has played on our bodies, life and world. In general, as an aromatherapist, I find it almost impossible to look at life in the usual jaded form anymore. With all my sense awareness tuned up, I sometimes feel as if the plants and their essential oils are communicating with me on many levels. I try to interact the same way with them. For example, I have persuaded plants to bloom by talking to them. I take joy from the many facets of their beauty — simply *looking* at colorful vegetables and fruit is a superbly enjoyable treat and actually eating one of them is a taste sensation.

However, I often go beyond the visible and tangible aspects of plants by trying to imagine their busy cells actually *creating* essential oils and putting them up for safekeeping. Often, I focus on my personal reaction to a plant and use what my intuition tells me when I'm selecting oils for my clients. When I apply the oils to my own skin I feel as though the vibrational current from the oils are mingling with my electrical aura to form a protective and healthy cocoon for my body.

* * * *

You might wonder, with all the horrible things going on in the world, "How can we think about something that seems as light-weight or nonsensical as scented therapy? Isn't it just another beautiful people fad?" You also may have to overcome that thought ingrained in the American psyche that says if something tastes too good, smells too good, or feels too wonderful, it must be suspect! In fact, aromatherapy has much more to offer than many know. It is an age-old practice that is much more than the application of prettily scented oils that leave a body perfumed and relaxed.

Correctly practiced, aromatherapy can do many things such as: relieve aches and pains; uplift our spirits and consciousness; help us to become more relaxed both physically and mentally; clean up our air and surroundings so that we can clear up more allergies, breathe better, and produce healthier children; bring us back in touch with plants (so we can improve our diets with herbs, eat more vegetables and fruit); and simply enhance our overall quality of life.

What's the point of living on a very superficial, artificial, and aggressive level — downing badly cooked fast foods, inhaling and ingesting more and more synthetic chemicals, and suffering from numerous maladies and discomforts? We can achieve a healthier, more joyous existence by choosing from the cornucopia of riches that nature has to offer. Beauty, health and serenity surrounds each one of us, it is just waiting to be noticed. We only have to make an effort to reach out and embrace it. Practicing aromatherapy treatments is one way to do that.

When I teach my workshop, I seek to make it a personal, eye-opening experience for each student. I try to offer them a different, more intimate

and enjoyable way of learning. This is what I hope to do in this workbook and with my audiotape of the same name. I encourage you to unlock your senses and increase the depth and breadth of your view of the world.

* * * *

For centuries, humans have relied on the massive plant kingdom for our food and medicines. However, from the vast network of plant life, members of three botanical families seem to be very useful and preferred sources of food and cures throughout history. These families are: Rosaceae (the Rose family), Labiatae (the Mint family) and Umbelliferae (the Carrot family). Just glance at some of the relatives listed for each family and you will see an extensive, if incomplete, list with some surprising inclusions!

Now, let us continue our scented journey by examining some plants from different parts of the world and the essential oils that they produce. Turn on your sense awareness (or turn it up, as the case may be) and stroll along with me.

Some scents will be extremely familiar to you and will already be stored in your scent memory banks. Others might be new and will have to be programmed into your scent memory banks for future retrieval and comparison.

aromatic culinary sources

Our first stop will be a visit to some aromatic plants from aromatic culinary sources. While we do eat fruit and other aromatic herbs from this group, we aromatherapists *do not recommend* ingesting any of these essential oils. They are medicines, not foods, and can actually be dangerous if you drink large quantities of them.

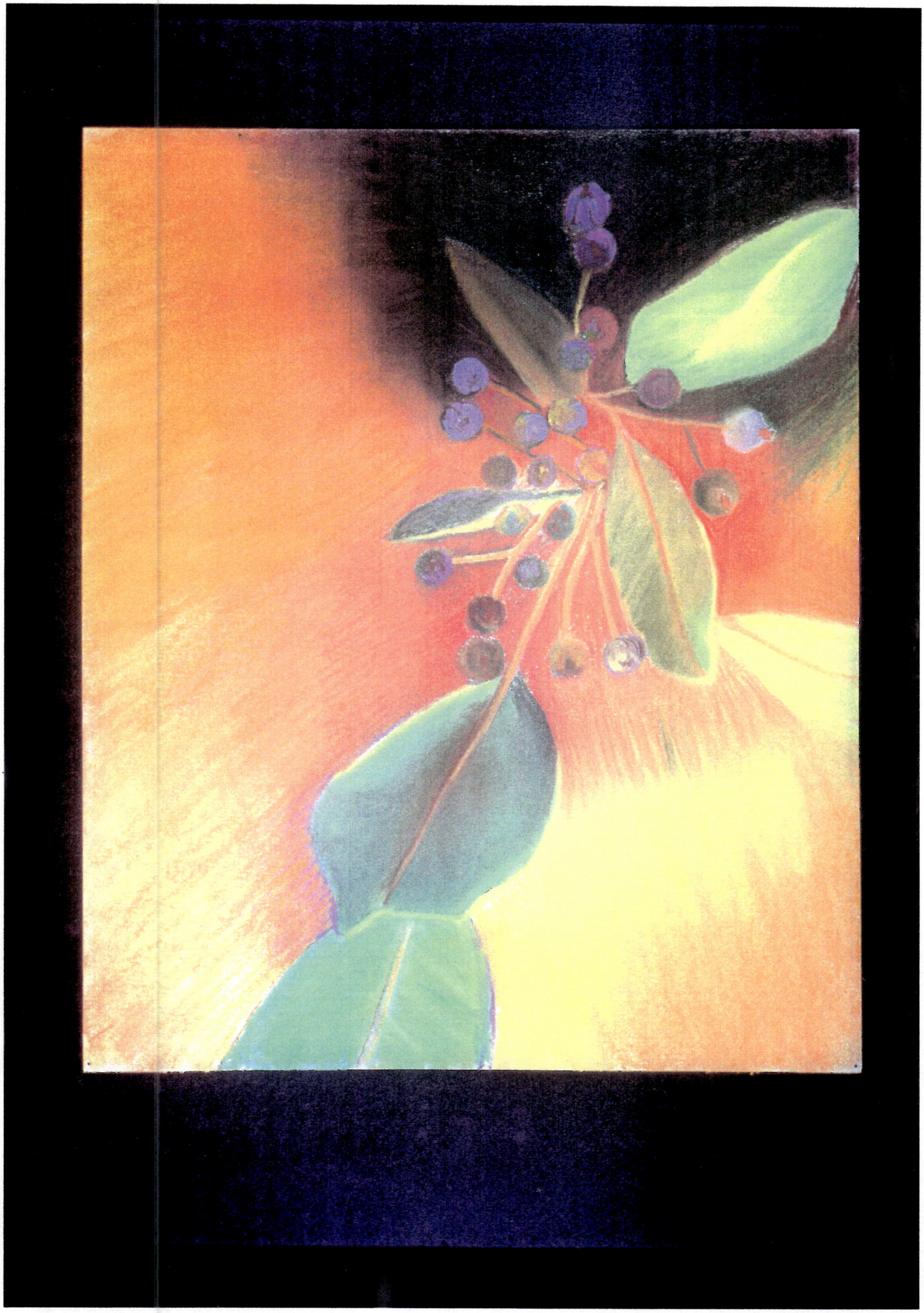

allspice

Its interesting cousins:

Clove
Eucalyptus
Myrtle Cajuput
Tea Tree

Applications:

circulation of legs
baths
sports pains
stimulation

Color of essential oil: russet

INSERT: essential oil

allspice

Imagine that you are in the lush green forests of the New World. Feel the warm breezes. Inhale the highly scented air that you can almost taste, hear the noises of the insects and animals and let the sun play on your skin as you walk through the trees. Look around — see the magnificent tree (about 40 feet high) with the dark green leaves and small clusters of white flowers? That is the ***allspice*** tree. Look closely at the small, brownish-purple berries. They are dried and used as a spice or steam-distilled to produce the essential oil. The leaves of this tree can also be steam-distilled to produce pimento leaf oil. In fact, pimento is the preferred name for this tree in Jamaica, where I come from.

Now sniff the oil — smell its undefinable spicy, clove/pepper scent? This is definitely a tropical aroma.

To tune into the long history allspice has had with man, let us consider several images. Imagine yourself as a pirate fighting other pirates to claim the "Jamaica gold" of this tree! You would definitely need a hot bath with allspice oil to help soothe your injuries afterwards! Consider yourself an Arawak woman living years before the Europeans showed up, brewing pimento berry tea to help your infant's upset stomach. Or you might just be a modern-day professional with a painful, repetitive-motion shoulder injury that is just crying out for a massage with allspice oil. Use your imagination!

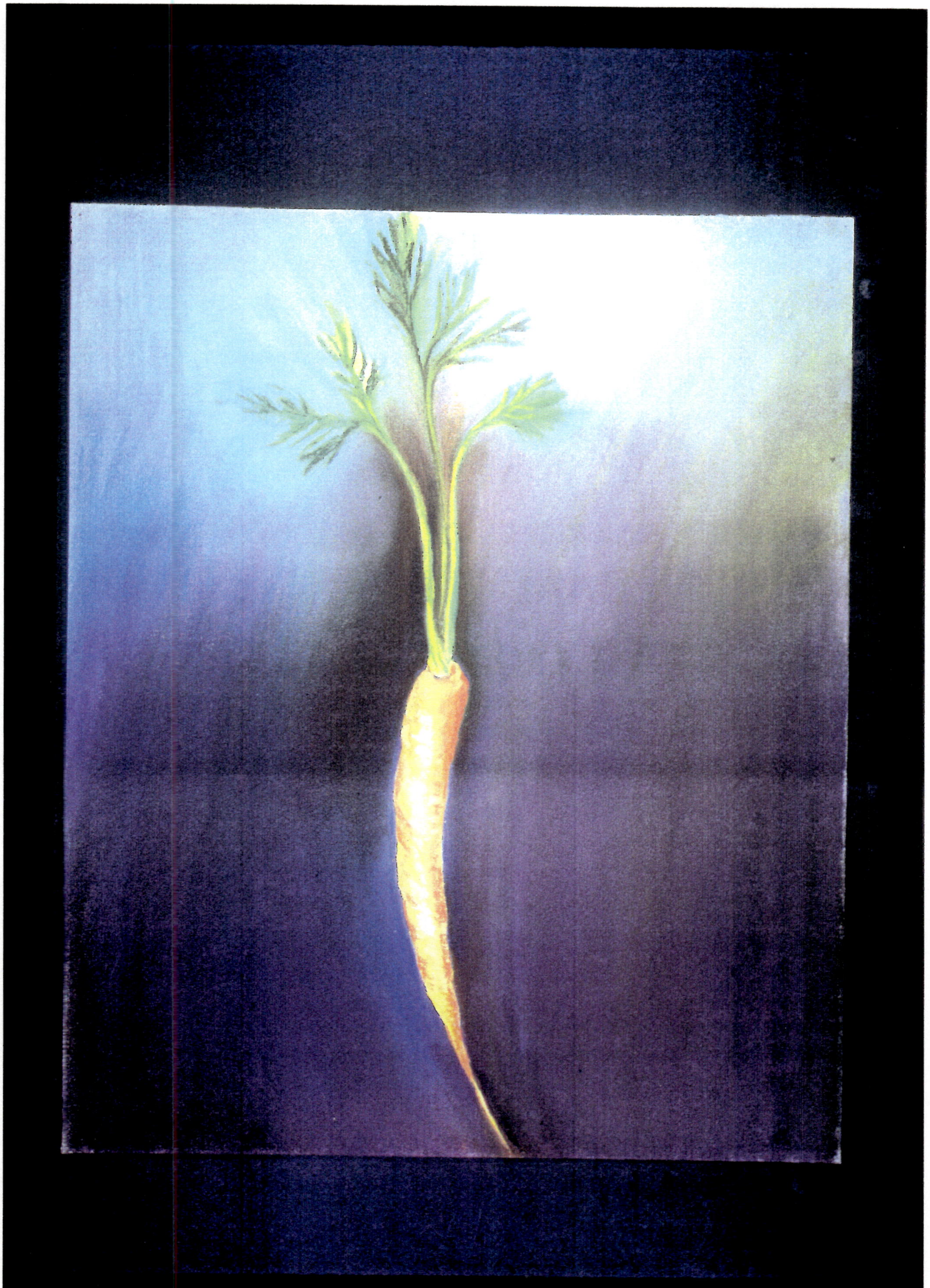

Umbelle ferae

carrot

Its interesting cousins:

Fennel
Coriander
Dill
Caraway
Angelica
Parsley
Anise
Galbanum
Hemlock
Parsnips

Applications:

sun tanning
skin care
sun damaged skin
blemishes
age spots
dry skin

Color of essential oil: orange

INSERT: essential oil

carrot

We wander back north to the temperate regions to meet a hardy survivor of the vegetable world. It is usually considered a fairly ordinary root that has been mandatory in filling soups and vegetable stews. But I think of it as the extraordinary ***carrot***!

Before it became so widely cultivated, the carrot's preferred growing places were ditches, fields, and by the roadsides. The modern carrot, a hybrid of various ancient carrots, seems to be just as hardy as its ancestors.

The interesting thing about carrots and man is the fact that we even thought to dig it up and look at the roots. The pale, fluffy umbel of flowers and stalks looks so airy and insubstantial that the discovery of the heavy orange-colored, sweet root must have been a welcome surprise! And beautiful indeed is the carrot plant with the root looking like a vertical shaft of light. The carrot, whether crunched raw, cooked, or juiced, is a very satisfying taste experience.

Carrot essential oil is distilled from wild carrot seeds and is orange-colored. Smell the oil — isn't it reminiscent of gasoline? Quite possibly it is the terpenes that produce this scent. On second sniff, the carrot scent emerges.

Picture yourself having the most beautiful skin in the world, protected from all of the harsh environmental elements. You can use the carrot oil with all of its carotenes to make your moisturizer, anti-wrinkle blend, or sun screen. Imagine mixing the luscious orange-colored oil with safflower or grapeseed oil and massaging it into your glowing, fresh face.

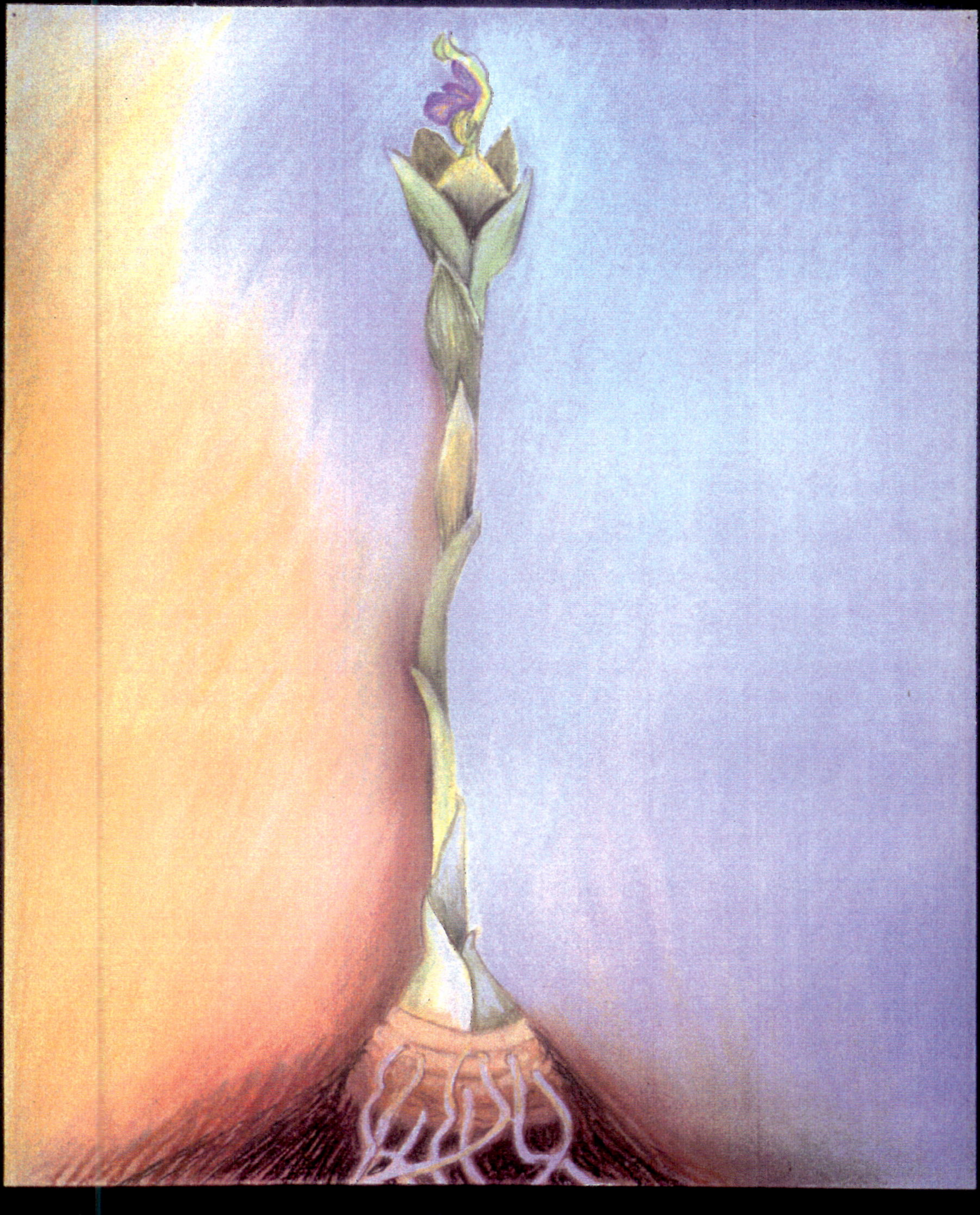

zingiberacea

ginger

Its interesting cousins:

Banana
Tumeric
Galangal
Guinea Grains
Zedoary

Applications:

warming
balancing
back aches
upset stomach
skin care

Color of essential oil: amber

INSERT: illustration of Ginger and essential oil

ginger

Now we are in tropical China looking over a field filled with stately-looking, erect green plants with yellow and purple flowers. This exquisite sentry also has hidden treasures.

Just below the ground some stems enlarge and spread out, filling themselves up with sugars and peppery carbon compounds to become the ***ginger*** rhizomes that we know and love. This spicy/sweet storage stem is dried and used as a garnish, in healing teas, or compresses by many people all over the world. Try a cup of hot ginger tea for colds, the flu or an upset stomach. The first thing that you might notice after drinking it is that you feel extremely hot and might even break into a sweat. This is because ginger is a febrifuge. Febrifuges elevate the body's temperature to encourage the cleansing of sweat. When we sweat we actually push out waste matter through the pores. Remember, the skin is the largest eliminatory organ of the body.

Steam distillation extracts the amber-colored essential oil from its rhizome. Sniff the oil — is it sweet, spicy or a combination of both?

Envision yourself as an ancient Chinese doctor willing your ill patient to recover with your ginger cures so you don't have to make restitution to the family. Or maybe you are in the tropics drinking Jamaican Ginger Beer for your upset tummy!

Imagine that sweet, warm scent combined as relaxing bath oil or massage oil. Try it by massaging it on your back or on your tummy for upset stomachs or backaches.

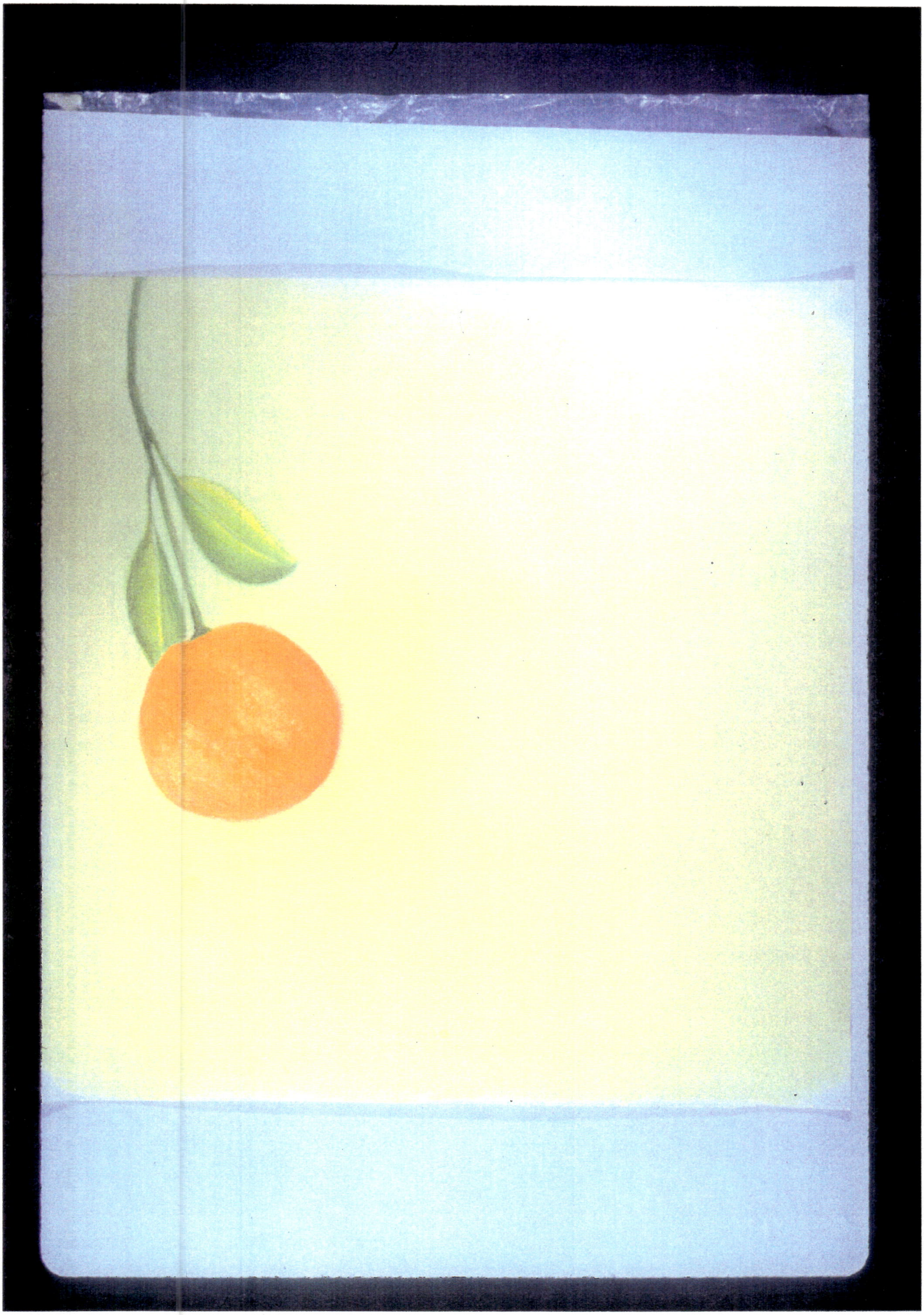

Rutaceae

orange

Its interesting cousins:

Buchu
Limes
Lemons
Jaborandi
Angostura
Bergamot
Tangerine
Prickly Ash
Rue
Wafer Ash

Applications:

skin care
insect repellant
relaxing
circulation
euphoria

Color of essential oil: orange

INSERT: essential oil

orange

Ah, here we are again, being bathed by friendly warm sunshine in southern climes. We are lying in a hammock swaying gently to and fro. Our eyes are closed. We are savoring the sweet, intoxicating air, and hearing the buzzing of insects. All around us are trees, most have shiny dark green leaves and are laden with luscious-looking fruit.

We reach up and pluck one of those globular fruits, peel it and eat it. The indescribable joy of eating a sweet ***orange*** fresh from the tree defies comparison with the taste of prepackaged juice. I consider this adventure the ultimate in languid sensuality. From the nose-tickling aroma of the peel to the actual taste of the citric fruit, to its round orange shape — I imagine that I am actually holding a miniature sun in my hands and eating its sunshine.

The orange is literally bursting with complex sugars and Vitamin C and the carotene principles which give it its color. Also vibrantly colored is the essential oil that is expressed from its rind.

Orange essential oil is excellent for all types of skin. It will introduce Vitamin C to the skin and circulatory system, relaxing and lubricating both. Imagine that you are working the healing energy of the sun's rays into your skin as you work the oil into your pores or as you relax in a bath improved with orange oil.

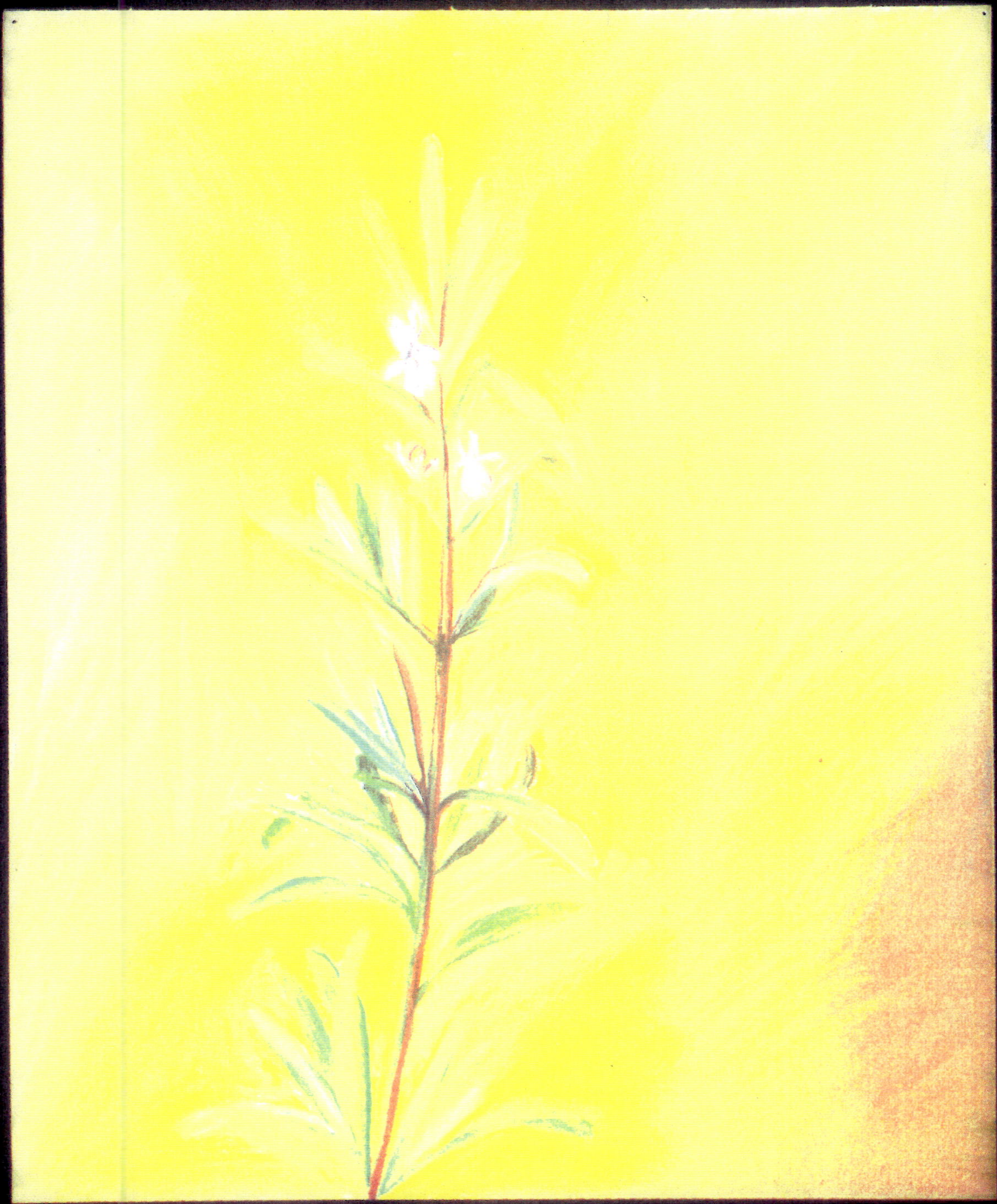

Labiatae

rosemary

Its interesting cousins:

Peppermint
Sage
Patchouli
Archangel
Melissa
Basil
Lavender
Spearmint
Hyssop
Pennyroyal
Savory

Applications:

decongestion
fluid retention
rejuvenation
hair growth
bruises
sprains
wounds
low blood pressure
arthritis

Color of essential oil: clear

INSERT: essential oil

rosemary

In the balmy Mediterranean region, not too far from the sea, originated a hardy, alley-cat survivor of the large mint family. This gutsy herbal bush welcomes the challenge of poor, sandy or chalky soil, but must have lots of sunshine to thrive.

The "rose of the Sea" or ***rosemary*** is now found all over the world, but let us examine it at its source again.

This evergreen shrub has thin, spiky, silverish leaves and may or may not be covered with tiny blue or white colored flowers in the spring. Now sniff the air around this bush. Notice the fresh, cool, piney scent? It is a refreshing and uplifting aroma that *stimulates* rather than sedates and *cools* the body instead of heating it up. This is the characteristic of herbs which originate north of the equator that separates them from the peppery, heating, co-working spices from south of the equator.

Now inhale rosemary again and feel your sinuses draining and fatigue lifting. Another scent emerges that sometimes tickles the taste buds in the back of the throat: camphor.

Steam distillation of the leaves yields the clear essential oil which we are now using for many ailments, from muscle injuries to fluid retention and sinus congestion.

Use the oil on hot, sticky summer days to cool the body down, while imagining you are strolling through the deserted streets of a small town in Greece or southern France. Just remember, however, that rosemary will elevate the blood pressure and should not be overused.

We now leave the aromatic kitchen section to explore other scented areas . . . .

Flower in the crannied wall,

I pluck you out of the crannies,

I hold you here, root and all, in my hand,

Little flower — but if I could understand

What you are, root and all, and all in all,

I should know what God and man is.

—*Flower in the Crannied Wall* by Alfred, Lord Tennyson

the flower garden

Come with me into my beautiful, imaginary and idealized flower garden. Close your eyes and inhale the symphony of scent that caresses your nostrils. Feel the various textures of scent —some warm, some hypnotic, some prickly, and others coolly sweet. Nature seems to have given flowers the widest orchestration of scent in the plant kingdom.

Imagine that through your mind's eye you look around, feasting on the sight of a multitude of colors in this garden. Isn't this a bonus of life? Doesn't it make you want to do a dance of life?
Feel deeply the joy these colors bring.

Step into the garden to meet some of these beauties individually.

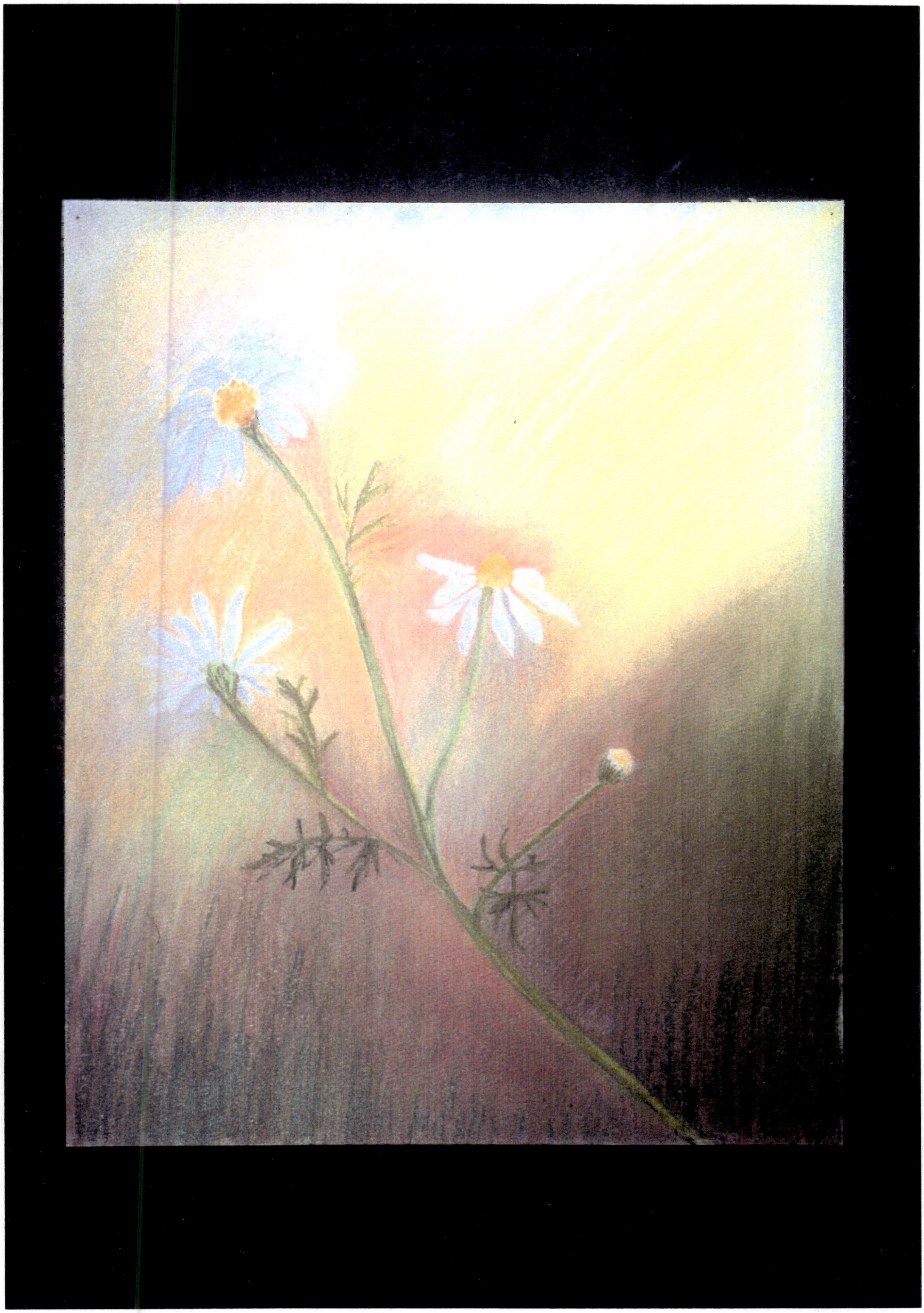

Compositae

chamomile

Its interesting cousins:

Arnica
Daisy
Dandelion
Marigold
Sunflower
Safflower
Yarrow
Tansy
Echinacea
Goldenrod
Boneset
Cornflower
Lavender Cotton
Mayweed

Applications:

skin care
couperose
under eye bags
relaxing babies
"female" problems
arthritis

Colors of essential oil: greenish/blue, blue

INSERT: essential oil

chamomile

See that daisy-like flower that looks like ground cover? Walk over to that area and smell a sweet, greenish-apple scent. We are walking on ***chamomile***, of which there are many varieties. All the varieties have flowers with fluffy yellow centers that are large in relation to the ring of tiny white petals that surround them. In Europe of long ago, chamomile was used as a fragrant ground carpet for many a stately home. Imagine you are walking on chamomile for some such home, stamping and walking on it to encourage the plant to spread. Now picture yourself in ancient Egypt at a ceremony where the priests are dedicating this flower to the Sun God, Ra. Let us hold up a bouquet of these daisies to the sun while asking Ra to bless our endeavors on Earth.

We return to our modern times to examine the flowers again. The flower itself has a musty aroma, but the leaves have a certain apple-like scent. That apple-like scent is transferred to the essential oil of the ***Roman Chamomile***, while the musty scent is transferred to the ***German Chamomile*** oil.

Now, dilute this oil in a vegetable oil base and massage it into your skin, imagining that the liquid calcium it contains is soothing your frazzled nerve endings and relaxing your body. This is an excellent oil for the whole family.

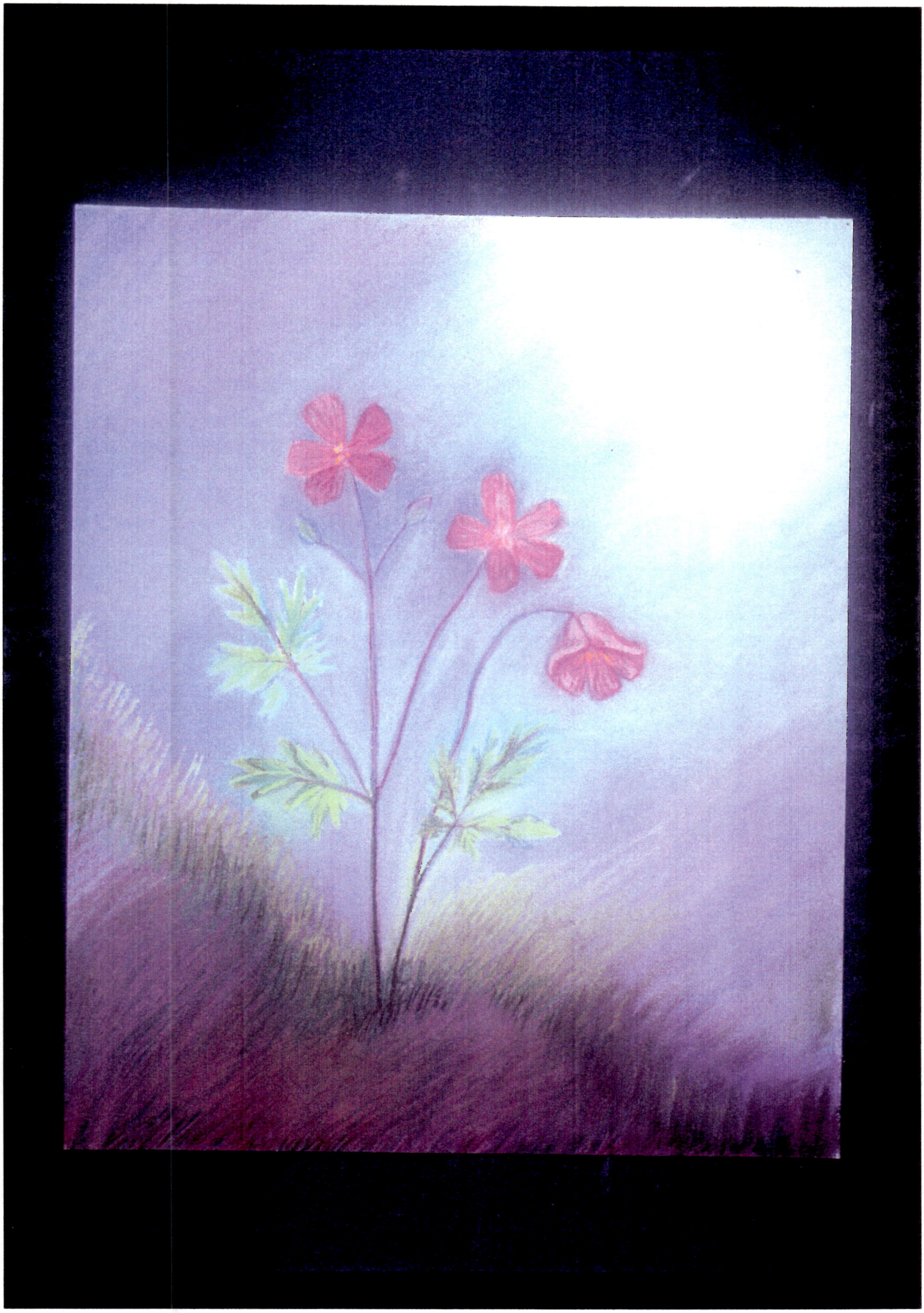

Geranium

herb robert

Its interesting cousins:

Cranesbills
Scented Geraniums

Applications:

dry skin patches
cracked skin
dermatitis
circulation tonic
wound healing
warm-up
(not recommended for sensitive complexions)

Color of essential oil: pale greenish

INSERT: essential oil

herb robert

Imagine your window boxes in the summer filled with bright red, pink or white Geraniums. Was there ever a more welcome sign of summer than these lovely, showy plants?

Now, meet their more interestingly medicinal cousin — the ***Herb Robert Geranium.*** The scented geraniums originated in South Africa and are now cultivated world-wide. Their hardier cousin, Herb Robert Geranium, is found growing wild in ditches, woods, rubbish heaps and on walls in such diverse countries as Britain, North and South America and North Africa.

Let's search my special garden for this plant. Yes, there it is by that earth wall — it has delicate, reddish stalks that are quite hairy with lovely, willowy fan-shaped leaves and fuchsia-colored, little flowers. As we approach Herb Robert, we see some little pod shaped bulbs with an erect stamen. That bulb and stamen identifies it as a member of the Cranesbill family. People in the olden days thought the bulb looked like a bird's long bill and named the plant accordingly.

The scent of this plant is quite rosy with a peppery tinge, as you might find when you sniff the essential oil. The oil is extracted from steam distillation of the whole plant and is greenish in color.

Let's travel backward in time to see how then ancients might have used infusions of this plant. We could be Cherokees washing our hair with this liquid or maybe using it as a wound healer. A continent away in Merrie Olde England, we could be wealthy gluttons suffering from the effects of fatty foods and take the infusion to help cure our hemorrhoids.

Nowadays, we can just use the oil as our ancestors used the plant. Say you pricked your finger on a thorn, let us dot some geranium oil on that cut and watch it clot within seconds. See? Or, maybe you stayed outside in the cold for too long and got overly chilled. A quick rub with diluted geranium oil will make you feel warm and cozy within minutes.

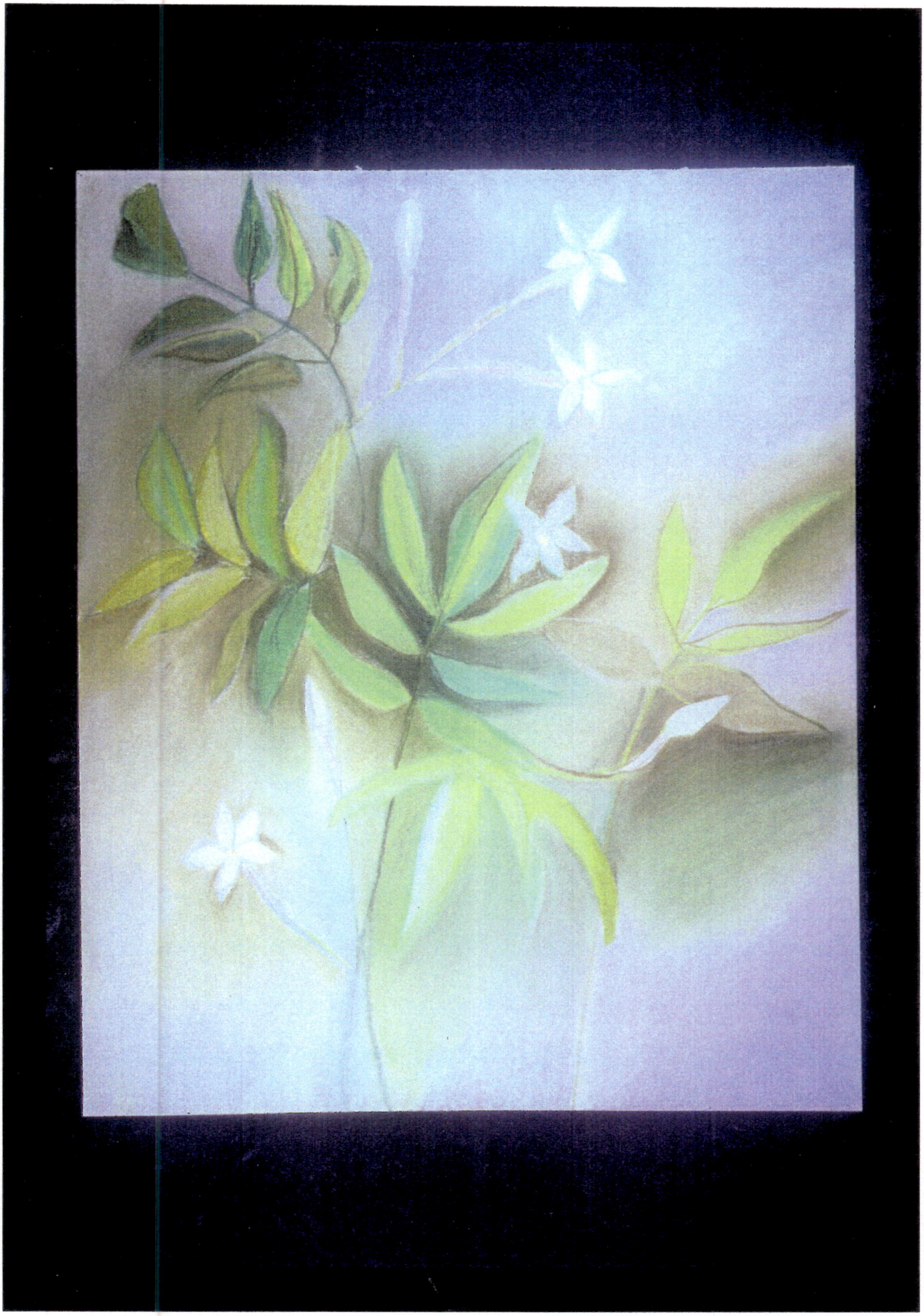

Oleaceae

jasmine

Its interesting cousins:

Olive
Ash
Lilac
Privet
Snowdrop Tree
Manna

Applications:

aphrodisia
acne
oily skin
uplifting
mood balancing
relaxing

Color of essential oil: honey amber to deep brown

INSERT: essential oil

jasmine

Ah, now we come to one of the loves of my life — that climbing bush with the pointed leaves and tubular-shaped, white, waxy flowers — the beloved ***jasmine***.

Originating in places like ancient Persia and Northern India, this plant is not truly tropical because it needs slightly cool temperatures and sheltered sun. In spite of its correct classification, it so reminds me of the tropics and Jamaica. I always want to stop and savor it, inhale its aroma, and reminisce while putting the blossoms in my hair.

I find the scent of these fresh flowers literally intoxicating. Interestingly enough, the dried flowers retain not *one iota* of that beautiful, honey-like aroma, but, rather, smell somewhat like hay.

That signifies how important it is to gather the fresh blossoms for oil extraction at just the right time. It also helps explain the expense of the oil. A notoriously resistant flower, the jasmine does not give up its essential oil to any old steam, but only to an exact blend of fats or in a chemical solvent.

Let's pretend we are courting in ancient Persia. As the young woman, we oil our hair carefully, then insert the jasmine flowers into our hair as we braid it. As the young gallant, we might insert the flower into our garments or bring a delightful posy for our loved one. What a lovely way to start a relationship!

If we believed in the African gods, we might implore the African goddess Oshun to make our sought-after-one our beloved by executing a ritual with jasmine oil.

I usually get goofily poetic trying to describe my reaction to the scent of jasmine. Go ahead, sniff the oil and make up your own sonnets!

See if jasmine doesn't make you smile, make you less stressed, and make you feel prettier! Rub the silky oil into your cheeks and watch them blossom. Or put a few drops in your bath and emerge, like Venus, a love goddess.

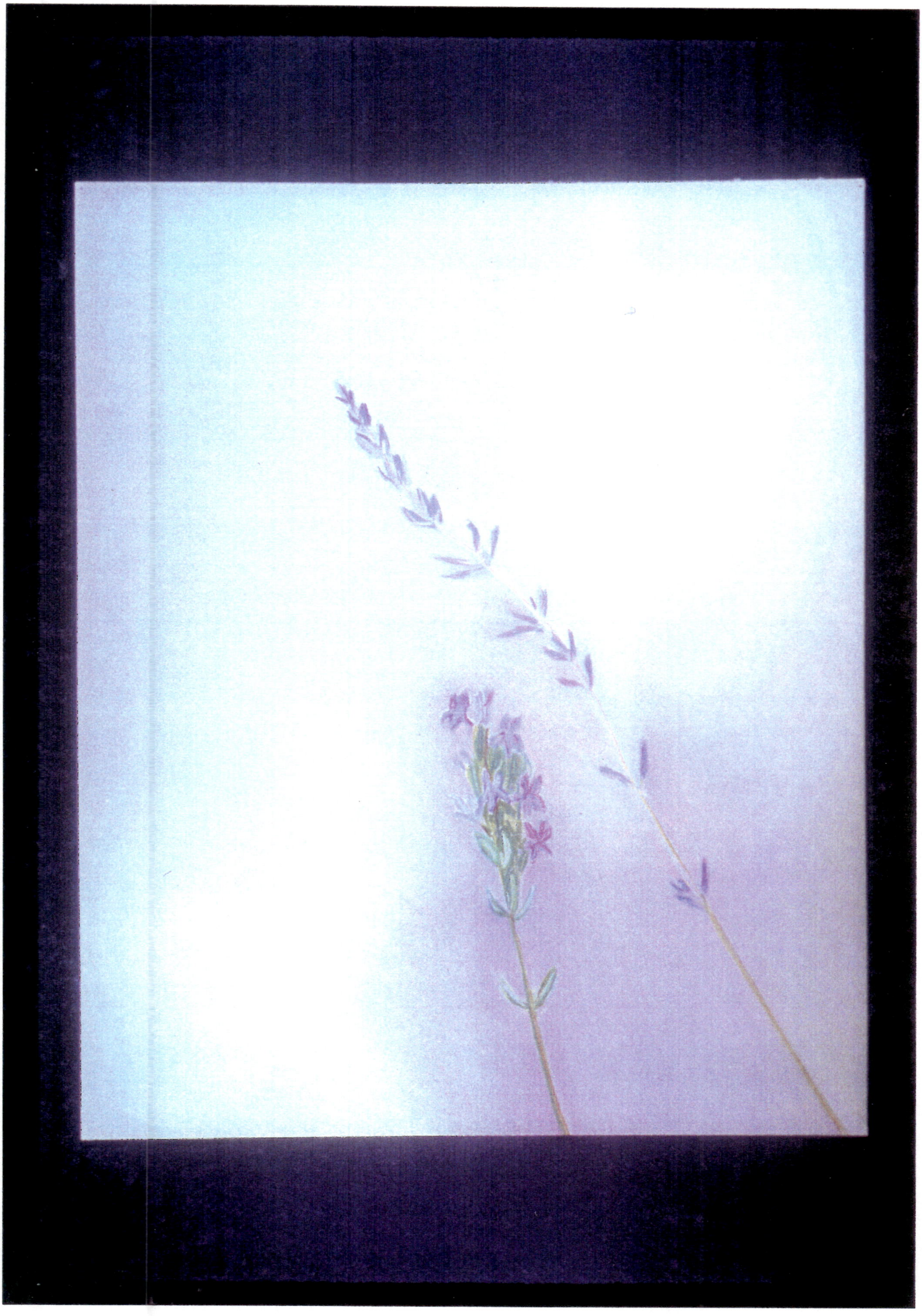

Labiatae

lavender

Its interesting cousins:

- Hemp Nettle
- Motherwort
- Horehound
- Marjoram
- Catnip
- Sage
- Thyme
- Rosemary
- Coleus

Applications:

- skin toning
- acne
- complexion care
- sprains
- wound healing
- decongestion
- insomnia
- insect repellent
- migraines

Color of essential oil: clear

INSERT: essential oil

lavender

As we continue to stroll in my garden, a color beckons us over. Oh, that pale purple color is a feast for the eyes. To see fields of blue on a hot summer's day is really one of life's many bonuses. Don't you feel cooler just looking at those beautiful ***lavender*** florets? Even if only in our imaginations, this sight can transport us to the fields of southern France. All we might need is a big picture hat, a folding chair, and an easel to complete the picture.

Lavender is also such a heavenly color that gazing at it can sometimes produce a high.

Let us sniff the wonderful air around the plants. Doesn't the aroma smell clean and fresh? Doesn't it make you want to take deeper, huge breaths? Lavender, probably a bit more than other essential oils, encourages us to take relaxing, deep breaths. The lavender affects this movement moderated by our stretch reflex, which is the arc that goes from our lungs to our brain. This reflex ensures that an out-breath is always followed by an in-breath.

Lavender has been popular for centuries and is used in many ways. Many add it to the wash (as an antiseptic as well as a cleanser), wear it as an insect repellent, and apply it for headaches. I'm sure there are few who have never used this wonderful herb.

The essential oil is steam-distilled from the whole lavender plant. You would think the oil should be a glorious lavender color, but it is, instead, an anti-climatic clear or yellowish color. This might be because the essential oil is actually made in the leaves and stalks and then sent to the flowers for storage.

One almost sure-fire remedy for restlessness or insomnia is a drop of pure lavender oil on the pillow before going to sleep. However, clients report that their wonderful, deep sleep is then punctuated by mysterious and awesome dreams.

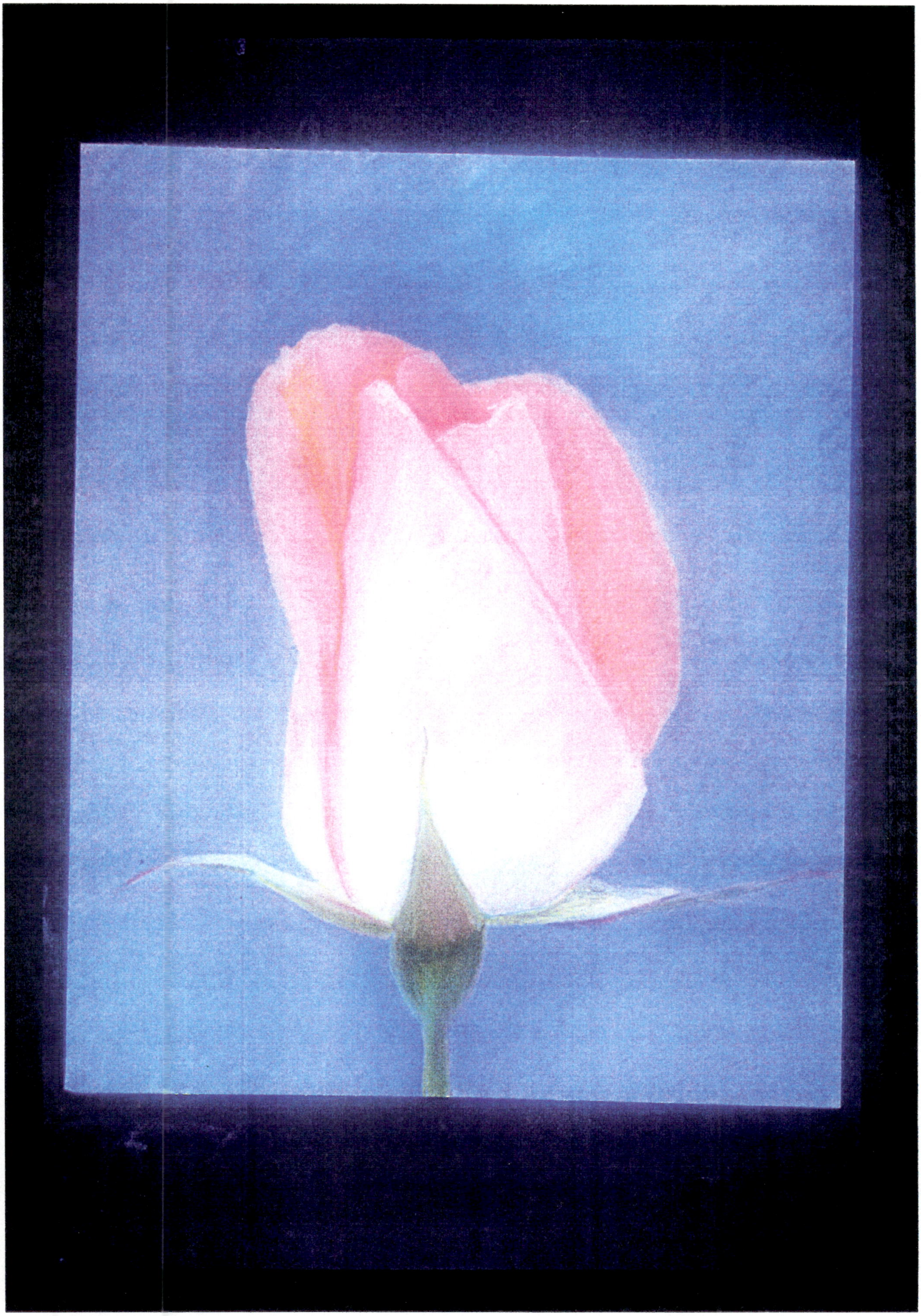

Rosacea

rose

Its interesting cousins:

Almond
Strawberries
Plum
Quince
Dogwood
Raspberries
Aquimony
Black Cherry
Dog Rose
Meadow Sweet
Blackberry
Peach
Soap Bark

Applications:

uplifting
complexion care
hangovers
aphrodisia
relaxing
"female complaints"
anxiety

Color of essential oil: greenish yellow

INSERT: essential oil

rose

Now we approach another love of my life, a flower so tampered with and hybridized by man that by rights it ought to have lost some of its allure, its mystery and its purity. Instead, it just seems to adapt to its new varieties of color, shapes and sizes with charming, glowing acceptance throughout the centuries.

Of course, I am waxing on about our beautiful friend, the ***rose***. The mass appeal of the rose cannot be dismissed or, I think, overstated. Who among us has not received a bouquet of roses without succumbing even momentarily to the romance of this gift? Doesn't the sight delight our eyes? Don't we want to bury our face in its blossoms? Didn't our heart give a slight jump at the meaning behind the gesture?

Some of us use rosewater in desserts, others eat rose petals in jams, and we can also thank the Dog Rose for the Vitamin C extracted from its Rose Hips.

Since there is something overwhelmingly feminine about the rose, some great ladies have claimed it as their own. So, let us imagine we are hanging out with Cleopatra, cruising the Nile on her barge. There are masses of rose petals on the floor, seats, and in our hair — everywhere! In fact, the less fortunate ones on the river banks can smell our barge long before we arrive. Truly, we are feeling no pain! The rose petals act as wings for our spirit and send it flying!

Since there are so many types of roses, the aroma of the essential oils can vary quite widely, from the citric ***Bulgarian Rose*** to the sweet ***Moroccan Rose.*** Sniff the ***Moroccan Rose*** sample and try to identify its complexity. Note its fairly dark color.

No matter what the rose essential oils smell like, they all leave your complexion with a "rosy glow" and a tender feel. You may also feel your anxieties melting away as you continue to massage it into your skin and inhale the aroma.

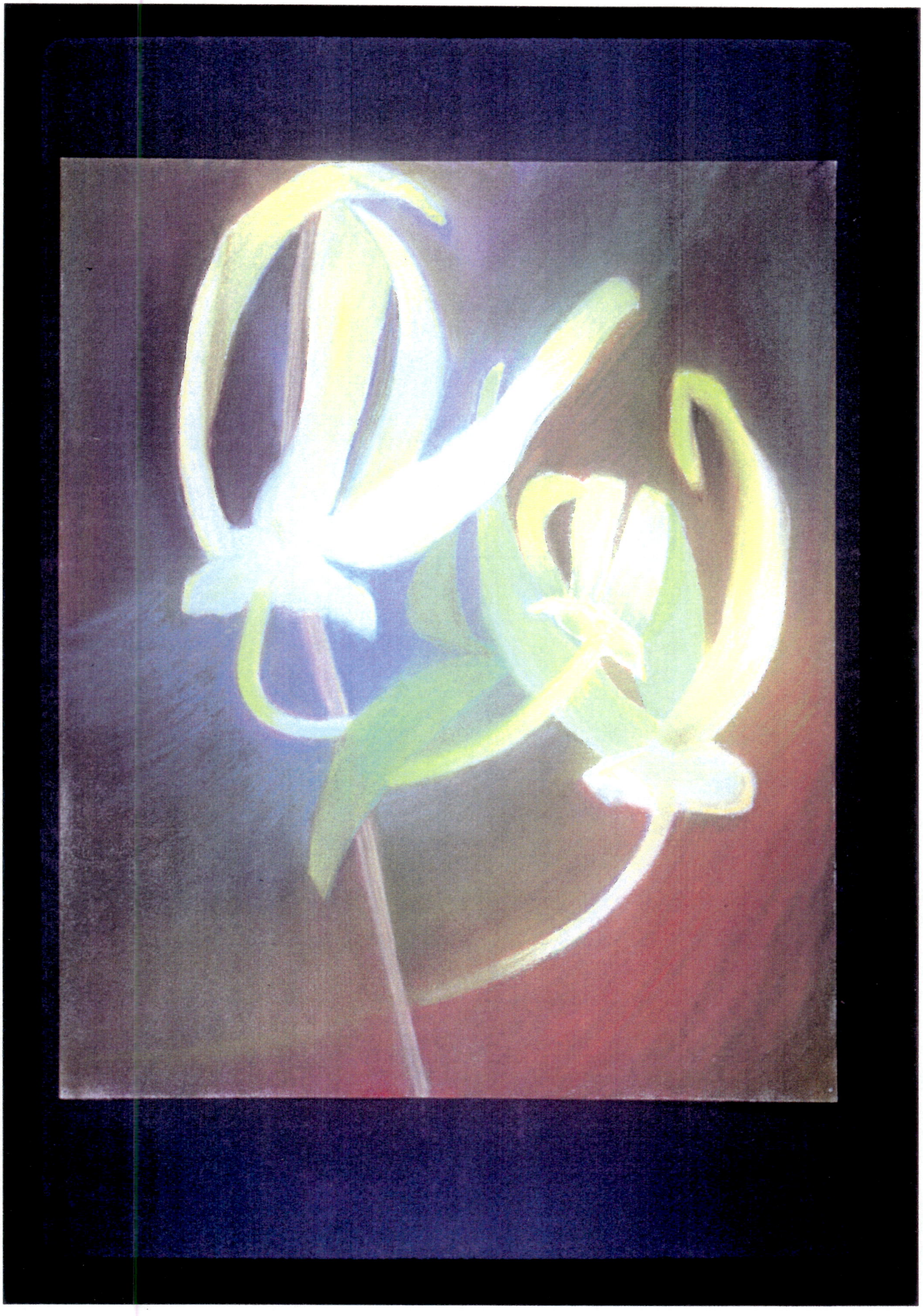

Anonceae

ylang-ylang

Applications:

- acne
- insomnia
- anxiety
- aphrodisia
- relaxation
- high blood pressure

Color of essential oil: greenish yellow

INSERT: essential oil

ylang-ylang

We are now at the edge of my garden walking toward some trees from different parts of the world.

The first tree is about 20 or 30 feet high and has glossy oval-shaped bright green leaves. Look at the blossoms. The small, tubular flowers grow in clusters and can be a strange color for a flower — greenish or pink. This is the ***ylang-ylang*** (pronounced "eelang eelang") tree, native to the Malaysian islands, but also found in many other countries.

The aroma of the flower is an intoxicating, jasmine-like syrup with the appeal of an aphrodisiac.

Let us go to the Philippines to participate in a tradition there. We are collecting ylang-ylang flowers and the rose-like sampaguita buds. Let's interlock the long shape of the ylang-ylang with the round buds of the sampaguita as we sew together our own beautiful and heady lei. Isn't that nice around our necks, or as a crown for our heads?

The essential oil is a greenish-yellow color and is extracted by steam distillation from the flowers. What does the aroma remind you of? Some say cough syrups, others say frangipani and still others detect cleaning fluid!

A very relaxing oil, ylang-ylang will calm an anxious heart in small doses, but increase anxiety in larger doses. This maybe because of its reputation of lowering blood pressure, so don't overuse it.

The silky feel of this oil makes it a pleasure to work with but I usually combine it with a citrus oil to overcome what I perceive as its less-than-wonderful scent.

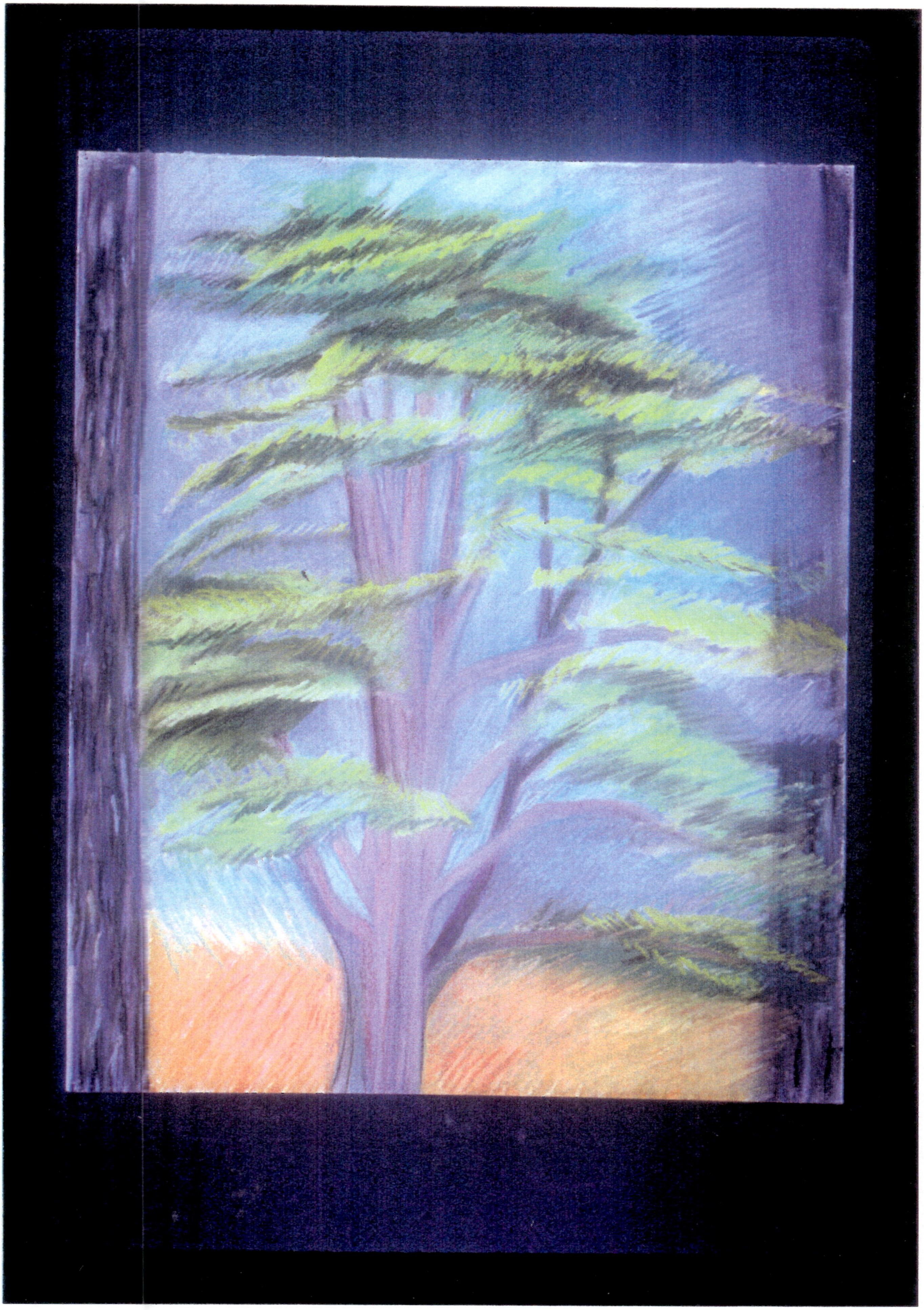

Conifer

cedarwood

Its interesting cousins:

Pine
Fir
Spruce
Larch
Cypress

Applications:

acne
scalp care
relaxation

Color of essential oil: amber

INSERT: essential oil

cedarwood

Let's go back in time to ancient Lebanon, Egypt and northeastern Africa. In the mountains stands these massive conifers — the ***cedarwood*** trees. A symbol of longevity and greatness, we value the fragrant wood for its perfume and also for building our boats, temples and coffins, and embalming our dead.

Shall we travel along with Queen Sheba of Ethiopia and her entourage to establish a trading cooperative with King Solomon of Israel? Maybe we will be there when her "black and comely" beauty bewitches him, along with her signature scent of "cedar of Lebanon" and honeyed fruit.

Or, maybe we can be workers helping to build the massive Temple of Solomon in Jerusalem, for God. The glossy, aromatic wood is extremely heavy to work with, but is a scent pleasure.

Consider the lure of this tree. It is massively and majestically rooted in the earth, but it grows higher and higher, firmly pointing towards the heavens. Many of these trees are still around, having been alive for thousands of years. They are truly the symbol of immortality that man has craved for himself; huge and solid figures, making us seem puny and insignificant in comparison. If we were to use the wood or its perfume might we become more conscious of secrets linking heaven and Earth?

Indeed, the scent of cedarwood oil can both uplift and relax the brain, before travelling downward to settle our stomachs. All the while it helps us to become more rooted or stable in our emotional balance.

Being a very calming oil, cedarwood relaxes an anxious heart, is wonderful for meditation or insomnia, and lends a comforting, woodsy note to overly sweet or floral blends.

We get the rich amber-colored oil through steam distillation of the wood chips.

* * * *

We have now left my ideal garden for now. I hope you've enjoyed visiting it with me and that you will make many return trips.

author's notes

During the 17 years I have been experimenting with essential oils, they never have ceased to amaze me. I feel that in some ways they are always communicating with me, as I have said before. During pre-treatment consultations with clients, it almost feels as if some oils jump into my consciousness saying, "choose me, choose me!" Most of the time this pushiness of the oils works — in fact, a good 95% of the time, I think. However, one memorable time when I was, for whatever reason, inspired to choose to combine fennel, eucalyptus, lily of the valley and patchouli as a massage oil for a particular client, it smelled so spectacularly bad when applied to the skin that I could imagine my poor client days later thinking "What is that smell?"

Despite these occasional lapses in communication, essential oils and I remain firm friends. As with friends, I have come to know certain quirky, interesting characteristic of these oils. For example, I remember telling my students that regular use of the oils can sometimes open up psychic awareness. One of my students, Mary, decided to take this as a challenge. When she got to her client's back as she was doing the massage she thought "Let's see if this works. I want you to think about flying — if you had wings, you could fly right now." And then she finished up her treatment. Afterwards, as she and the client were chatting through the post-treatment consultation, she casually asked if there was anything different about the treatment than those she had previously given. The client immediately said "funny you should ask. When you were doing my back, I had the strangest sensation that I wanted to fly!" What do you think of that, then?

Another thing I have noticed is that essential oils (still in their unopened bottles) will substantially cool down the surrounding air. Perfume and fragrance oils, on the other hand, will heat up the surrounding air — sometimes to the point of being overwhelming. There have been many times that I've done trade fairs in hot, airless rooms, and my booth was the one cool, fragrant oasis in the place. People had no trouble finding my booth and would gravitate to it to refresh themselves!

Now, do I think aromatherapy might be one of the answers for serious diseases? I don't know. My work with cancer and AIDS patients has been patchy and inconsistent. The clients that were recommended to me just couldn't believe aromatherapy massage could be of any use to them. As a result, they either didn't show up for their appointments, or only had one. I do believe, however, that in the hands of caring holistic doctors, essential oils could offer a dramatic turning point in the quality-of-life for very ill patients. I would direct doctors so interested to read the detailed texts of Rene Maurice Gattefosse in which he discusses his usage of essential oils in hospitals with tubercular patients and notes the encouraging results he observed.

On the other hand, my regular clients have come in from time to time with a wide range of diseases that were markedly improved after the essential oils got to work helping all the systems (especially the lymph) to self-cleanse and tone. Now, the majority come to help maintain good health — sort of like a tune up — and to discourage stress-related problems. And they show marvelous results on their medical examinations.

* * * *

It's very important when giving regular aromatherapy treatments to work in a well-ventilated room. The essential oils have such a strong detoxifying capacity that the toxins that they pull out of the body through the pores can fill the room after a treatment. This bad air is especially noticeable if the client is ill, eats a lot of meat or cheese, or drinks/smokes a lot. You must clear this air out between clients or you might leave yourself depleted — you can absorb the poisons in the air very rapidly during your work. In fact, sometimes you can taste the stale air in the back of your throat at the end of your treatment. To speed up the cleansing of the air, burn ordinary beeswax candles (not incense or smudge sticks).

This extreme cleansing afforded by the first aromatherapy treatment can be quite painful for the client if s/he is ill, extremely stressed or muscle bound. Each subsequent treatment, however, becomes noticeably less painful and more blissful.

* * * *

I'll leave you now by creating for you two special oils: Morning Glory (Good to be Alive Blend) and Nighttime Peace.

MORNING GLORY

5 drops Orange Blossom Oil
20 drops Lavender Oil
5 drops Jasmine Oil
5 drops Black Pepper Oil
10 drops Pine Oil
10 drops Pettigrain Oil

Add the oils to 1 oz. of Safflower Oil, mixing well. Use either of the following ways: pour 2 capfuls in a set bath; or pour some of this blend on a washcloth, rub into feet and stand on this washcloth while showering; or vigorously massage blend into skin after showering.

NIGHTTIME PEACE

10 drops of Lavender Oil
10 drops of Cedarwood Oil
10 drops of Orange Oil

Mix together in a small glass vial. Put one drop on a tissue and inhale constantly before retiring. Or put one or two drops on your pillow before going to sleep.

Gather ye rosebuds while ye may
Old time is still a-flying;
And this same flower that smiles to-day,
Tomorrow will be dying....

— Robert Herrick

I saw eternity the other night,
Like a great ring of pure and endless light,
All calm, as it was bright,
And round beneath it time in hours, days, years,
Driven by the spheres
Like a vast shadow moved, in which the world
And her train were hurled.

— Henry Vaughn

conclusion

Now, sadly, we leave our enchanted aromatherapy world of botanicals and specialized scenarios. However, you can revisit this world many times over by re-reading this workbook or playing the audiotape. I do hope this workbook has opened up for you new and different ways of approaching aromatherapy. Your own personal interpretation of the oils, their combinations and how to use them is very important. But study, practice and communication with other aromatherapists is also vital if you wish to become a master in this field.

If you would like a more exciting challenge to help you increase your personal sense awareness, use the exercises I have discussed as a jumping off point — go on to create your own scenarios around other plants and other situations. Don't let anything limit your imagination and desire to learn. I encourage you to explore this exquisite science. Seek out trained aromatherapists for treatment and start using the oils every day. Pleasant surprises await you.

There are many different ways of experiencing life, of interpreting ideas and practicing our craft. Each aromatherapist has his or her own personal view of each of these large issues and how they relate to each other. To me, the most important elements to remember are the purity of intent, the interconnectedness of life, and the importance of the spirit.

In addition to these more cerebral and spiritual aspects of aromatherapy practice, we must also keep in mind the reality of the physical body that we are affecting with our treatments and how it operates. Health is normal for our bodies. Our bodies usually do a good job of maintaining their own healthy balance with little conscious attention on our part. Essential oils, being a very potent part of plant medicines (from which modern medicine sprang), seem to help our physical systems maintain this healthy balance that they strive for naturally. Regular massage with the oils can help to discourage colds, the flu and other infectious diseases; sooth arthritis pain; reduce fluid retention; eliminate waste deposits; help skin care problems; aid with wound healing; encourage a more peaceful frame of mind; and cure many, many other ailments.

Relaxation therapy is another way to encourage blissful healing and spiritual awareness. Most aromatherapists treat their clients with aromatherapy massage, combining the use of medicinal extracts with relaxation, or massage therapy to improve both the patient's cosmetic and spiritual well-being. This multilevel approach to health may help explain why people that receive regular aromatherapy massages look as if they've discovered the fountain of youth!

* * * *

Holistic health, meditation, aromatherapy, religious science and the like are all different pathways leading to the same goal: unlocking spiritual pathways that naturally lead to the search for the return journey home to God.

list of aromatherapy suppliers

E-Scentially Yours, The Aromatherapy Place

24 East 38th Street
New York, NY 10016
212-545-0229

The Essential Oil Company (Professionals Only)

Robert Seidel
P.O. Box 206
Portland, OR 97034
503-697-5992

Philip Samuel (Indfrag Private, Ltd.)

S-913, Manipal Centre
Dickenson Road
Bangalore 560 042 India
0812-589521

Richard Taylor

50 New Street, P.O. Box 93
Port of Spain, Trinidad
809-625-2580

bibliography

Ackerman, Diane. *A Natural History of the Senses* (New York: Random House, Inc., 1990)

Anthony, Catherine Parker & Thibodeau, Gary A. *Anatomy and Physiology* (St. Louis, MO: C.V. Mosby, Co., 1979)

Arctander, Steffan. *Perfume and Flavor Materials of Natural Origin* (Elizabeth, NJ: by author, 1960)

Arnould-Taylor, William. *Aromatherapy* (London, England: Arnould-Taylor Education, Ltd., 1988)

Bonar, Ann. *Gardening for Fragrance* (London, England: Ward Lock, Ltd., 1990)

Curtis, Helena. *Biology* (New York: Worth Publishers, Inc., 1983)

Garland, Sarah. *The Complete Book of Herbs and Spices* (New York: The Viking Press, 1979)

Gerard, John. *The Herbal or General History of Plants, The Complete 1633 Edition revised by Thomas Johnson* (New York: Dover Publications, Inc. 1975)

Kamm, Minnie Watson. *Old Time Herbs for Northern Gardens* (London, England: Dover Publications, Inc., 1971)

Holum, John. *Elements of General and Biological Chemistry* (New York: John Wiley & Sons, Inc., 1983)

Lautie, Raymond. & Passebecq, Andre. *Aromatherapy* (London, England: Thorsons Publishers, Ltd., 1979)

List, P.H. & Schmidt, P.C. *Phytopharmaceutical Technology* (Boca Raton, FL: CRC Press, Inc., 1989)

Miller, Richard Alan. *The Magical & Ritual Use of Herbs* (Vermont: Destiny Books, 1983)

Potterton, David. Editor. *Culpepper's Color Herbal* (New York: W. Foulsham & Co., Ltd., 1983)

Ritchason, Jack. *The Little Herb Encyclopedia* (Orem, Utah: BiWorld Publishers, 1982)

Riva, Anna. *Golden Secrets of Mystic Oils,* (California: International Imports, 1978)

Robertson, Diane. *Jamaican Herbs* (Kingston, Jamaica: Jamaican Herbs, Ltd., 1982)

Robertson, Diane. *Live Longer, Look Younger with Herbs* (Kingston, Jamaica: Stationary & School Supplies, Ltd., 1990)

Rose, Jeanne. *Herbs & Things* (New York: The Putnam Publishing Group, 1972)

Sellar, Wanda. *The Directory of Essential Oils* (England: C.W. Daniel Co., Ltd., 1992)

Suskind, Patrick. *Perfume* (New York: Alfred A. Knopf, Inc., 1986)

Thomson, William A.R., Edited by. Schultes, Richard Evans. Revised by. *Medicines from the Earth* (Maidenhead, England: McGraw Hill Book Co. UK, Ltd., 1978)

Tissarand, Robert. *The Art of Aromatherapy* (England: C.W. Daniel Co., 1977)

Tisserand, Robert. Edited by. *Gattefosse's Aromatherapy* (England: C.W. Daniel Co., Ltd., 1937)

Valnet, Jean. *The Practice of Aromatherapy* (England: C.W. Daniel Co., Ltd., 1980)

Wren, R.C. *Potters New Cyclopaedia* (London: Potter's Herbal Supplies, Ltd., 1988)